NUTRITION FOR GOLDEN YEARS

A SENIOR'S GUIDE TO VIBRANT HEALTH

TABLE OF CONTENTS

Dedication

Preface

Introduction

Chapter 1: Senior Nutrition Essentials

Chapter 2: Building a Healthy Senior Diet

Chapter 3: Superfoods for Seniors

Chapter 4: Special Diets and Health Conditions

Chapter 5: Cooking and Meal Preparation

Chapter 6: Staying Active and Eating Right

Chapter 7: Overcoming Nutrition Challenges

Chapter 8: Dining Out and Social Eating

Chapter 9: Tracking Your Nutrition

Chapter 10: Embracing Vibrant Health in Your Golden Years

Conclusion

Additional Resources

DEDICATION

To all the golden souls who have graced our lives with wisdom, laughter, and love. This book is dedicated to you, our cherished seniors, who continue to inspire us with your resilience and zest for life. May your golden years be filled with vibrant health, nourishing meals, and the joy of each moment.

PREFACE

Welcome to the journey of a lifetime – your golden years. As the curtain rises on this new chapter of life, you are presented with a precious opportunity to savor every moment, relish each day, and embrace the many joys that come with aging gracefully.

However, the path to vibrant health in your golden years is not without its twists and turns. It requires understanding, adaptation, and a willingness to empower yourself with the knowledge and tools necessary to navigate the challenges and reap the rewards.

This book, "Nutrition for Golden Years: A Senior's Guide to Vibrant Health," is your compass on this journey. It's a guide designed to shed light on the ways nutrition can be your steadfast ally in achieving the quality of life you deserve. We will explore the transformation of nutritional needs as you age and uncover the key nutrients that support your health and well-being.

But this is not just a book about what to eat. It's a celebration of the art of living well in your golden years. It's about understanding the flavors and textures that make meals a delight, and it's about the joy that sharing food with friends and family can bring.

We will also venture into the territory of common health concerns that may require special dietary considerations. Whether it's heart health, managing diabetes, or addressing specific dietary restrictions, we'll provide guidance to ensure that health challenges do not hinder the pursuit of a vibrant life.

Furthermore, we'll explore the harmonious relationship between physical activity, nutrition, and weight management. Together, these elements will provide you with the vitality to seize every opportunity and experience the richness of life.

This book is not just a manual; it's a companion in your quest for health, happiness, and fulfillment. It's a resource that you can return to again and again, each time gaining new insights and inspiration.

So, as you embark on this journey, let "Nutrition for Golden Years" be your trusted partner. Dive into its pages with an open heart and a curious mind, and let it be your guide to vibrant health, nourishing meals, and a life well-lived.

With every chapter you explore, remember that it's never too late to rewrite the script of your life. It's never too late to savor the joys of your golden years. So, let's begin this journey together.

Bon appé tit and bon voyage to the vibrant and fulfilling years that lie ahead!

Warm regards,

Grace Ben-Council

Author

INTRODUCTION

Hello and welcome to "Nutrition for Golden Years: A Senior's Guide to Vibrant Health." This book is your travel companion while you work to age gracefully, emphasising the importance of a nutritious diet. Let's take a minute as we begin this inquiry to appreciate the significant significance of the decisions we make regarding the food we eat in our later years.

The Importance of Nutrition in Aging Gracefully

Ageing is a natural process that happens to everyone, and it can be a beautiful, satisfying, and enriching journey. It's a chance for us to enjoy the knowledge and experiences we've accumulated over the years. However, it's also a time when our bodies go through changes, so maintaining a healthy lifestyle, especially with regard to diet, is essential for ageing gracefully.

The impact of nutrition on the ageing process is truly astonishing. It can boost our vigour, promote our general health, and give us the chance to live each day to the fullest. What we eat has a direct impact on how we feel, how our bodies work, and how we enjoy our golden years.

In the chapters that follow, we'll delve into the fundamentals of senior nutrition, looking at how our dietary requirements vary as we get older, the most important nutrients for senior health, and the importance of creating a diet that promotes wellbeing in our later years.

We'll talk about senior-friendly eating recommendations, the value of moderation and being hydrated, as well as how to include superfoods in your diet to support ageing gracefully. You'll learn about special diets for prevalent medical issues like diabetes and heart disease, as well as simple, wholesome dishes created especially for seniors. You'll also get helpful meal-planning advice. We'll also stress the significance of the link between healthy diet and exercise, as well as age-appropriate weight management techniques.

We'll discuss promoting digestive health, dealing with changes in appetite and taste, and the potential role of supplements as we tackle typical issues in senior nutrition. We will discuss eating out, keeping healthy eating habits in social situations, using notebooks and apps to track your nutrition, and working with healthcare providers when necessary.

We'll end by urging you to adopt a senior lifestyle of vibrant health, embrace mindful eating, and set and meet your nutrition objectives.

As you enter your golden years, use this book as a resource to help you make educated and healthy food decisions. We will examine the options for ageing gracefully while promoting your bright health together. So let's start this exciting adventure together and pray for a fulfilling one that is full of health and vigour.

CHAPTER 1

SENIOR NUTRITION ESSENTIALS

It's vital to recognise that the nutritional decisions we make play a crucial role in this endeavour as we set out on our road to bright health in our golden years. This chapter is your first step towards understanding how your nutritional requirements change as you age and it highlights the most important nutrients for preserving your health and vigour.

Understanding How Nutritional Needs Change with Age

The natural and beautiful process of ageing comes with its own set of specific issues, particularly in terms of nutrition. Understanding how your body changes as you age is the key to ageing gracefully. Your body goes through a number of changes as you age.

Your metabolic rate gradually declining is one of the biggest alterations. This implies that less calories may be needed by your body to maintain your current weight and level of energy. It's important to keep in mind, though, that fewer calories do not necessarily mean more nutrition. This emphasises the significance of making sure every calorie you take is high in important nutrients. Your body is less tolerant of empty calories when your metabolism is slower, which emphasises the need for nutrient-dense foods that deliver the most advantages per mouthful.

With ageing, your digestive tract, which is a vital part of the complex process of feeding, also experiences changes. Some people can notice a decline in appetite, which might result in eating fewer meals during the day. This makes it even more important for each meal to provide your body with the vital nutrients it needs to operate at its best. The importance of your food decisions and the bioavailability of nutrients is further highlighted by the possibility that alterations to your gastrointestinal system can impact nutrient absorption.

Additionally, as you age, you can notice a loss in bone density and muscle mass. Here, the importance of nutrients like protein, calcium, and vitamin D is highlighted as they become even more crucial. Losing muscle can affect your metabolism and mobility, which emphasises the need for specialised nutrition to keep your body healthy and powerful.

Key Nutrients for Senior Health

Focusing on particular nutrients that are essential to your health and well-being can help you thrive in your golden years. These nutrients promote numerous facets of your health by serving as the building blocks of vitality:

1. Calcium: This mineral is necessary for keeping healthy bones and avoiding osteoporosis, which can cause brittle bones.

2. Vitamin D: This vitamin promotes bone health and helps the body absorb calcium. Additionally, it affects a number of other physiological functions, such as immune system operation.

3. Vitamin B12: Vitamin B12 is necessary for sustaining mental acuity and general health, as well as for cognitive function and nerve health.

4. Fibre supports digestive health, helps people manage their weight, and keeps blood sugar levels normal.

5. Antioxidants: Strong antioxidants include nutrients like the vitamins C and E. They combat inflammation and oxidative stress, two things linked to a number of chronic illnesses.

6. Omega-3 fatty acids are crucial for preserving a healthy heart and brain since they are known to improve heart health and cognitive function.

7. Protein: Protein is essential for maintaining general strength and muscle mass. It is essential for preserving mobility and an active lifestyle since it supports muscular function.

8. Folate: This B-vitamin helps to prevent some birth abnormalities and is essential for DNA

synthesis and cell growth.

9. Potassium: In addition to being crucial for controlling blood pressure, potassium helps to maintain healthy muscle function, which is necessary for overall mobility and vigour.

We will go more into these essential nutrients as we go along in this eBook, providing advice on how to successfully include them in your diet to promote your general wellbeing as you age.

The knowledge you will acquire from this book will serve as your guide to accepting nutrition as a crucial aspect of ageing gracefully. With the help of these realisations, you'll be more equipped to make decisions that will improve your health, energy, and the possibility of completely appreciating your later years. Let's thus proceed with our investigation of this path to bright health step by step.

CHAPTER 2

BUILDING A HEALTHY SENIOR DIET

This chapter, "Building a Healthy Senior Diet," is your guide to arranging a balanced and nourishing food throughout your senior years. throughout the symphony of life, our dietary choices create a melodic tune that reverberates throughout our well-being. We'll go over senior-friendly eating recommendations, the fine art of portion control, how often to eat, and the significance of hydration for preserving senior health.

Senior-Friendly Dietary Guidelines

A senior-friendly diet is made up of colourful, healthful ingredients that have been specifically chosen to meet the special requirements and preferences of people in their golden years. It is an appreciation of nutritious, nourishing foods that are delectable.

The first step in adopting a senior-friendly diet is including a range of foods from various dietary groups. This variety makes sure you get a wide variety of nutrients that are crucial for your health. Lean proteins, whole grains, fruits, vegetables, and healthy fats are a few of these. The fundamental vitamins, minerals, and nutrients that make up each dietary group are the cornerstones of good health.

You should concentrate on the following nutritional recommendations to create a diet that is senior-friendly:

1. Meals That Are Balanced: Strive to prepare meals that are nutritionally sound and contain a source of lean protein, complex carbohydrates, and healthy fats. Together, these components deliver enduring energy and satisfaction.

2. Colourful Plates: Include a range of colourful fruits and vegetables on your plate since they each contain antioxidants and phytonutrients that have their own unique health advantages.

3. Fiber-Rich Foods: The staples of your diet should include whole grains, legumes, and fibre vegetables. For healthy digestion, stable blood sugar levels, and weight management, fibre is crucial.

4. Limit your intake of highly processed and high-sugar foods, as these can have a negative impact on your health. Choose full, raw choices instead.

5. Eat mindfully by paying attention to your body's signals of hunger and fullness. Overeating can be avoided by eating consciously, which allows you to enjoy each meal.

6. Reduced Sodium Intake: Too much sodium raises blood pressure and causes other health problems. Pay attention to how much salt is in your diet and choose low-sodium options.

7. Healthy Cooking Techniques: Choose cooking techniques like steaming, roasting, and grilling that maintain the nutritional content of your

food and lessen your dependency on frying or cooking with excessive amounts of fat.

Portion Control and Meal Frequency

To ensure that you're giving your body the proper quantity of food to support your health and energy needs without overindulging, practise portion management. Because of a slower metabolism as we get older, we frequently need less energy. Portion control is therefore even more important.

Never forget that how much you eat is equally as important as what you eat. Smaller, portion-controlled meals can assist in preserving a healthy weight and avoiding calorie overconsumption.

Along with quantity control, meal frequency is important. Instead of three major meals throughout the day, think about replacing them with smaller, more frequent meals and snacks. This strategy can assist you in sustaining consistent energy levels throughout the day and preventing excessive hunger, which could result in unhealthy food selections.

Hydration and Senior Health

A crucial component of elder health is hydration. It's important to pay attention to your water needs as you age since your body may become less effective at detecting thirst. Numerous health problems, such as urinary tract infections, constipation, and diminished cognitive function, can be brought on by dehydration.

The general recommendation is to drink 8 to 10 cups (64 to 80 ounces) of water each day. Your particular requirements, though, might change depending on your exercise level, the weather, and your general health. Maintaining sufficient hydration requires paying attention to your body's cues, such as dry mouth or dark urine.

We will continue to look at how to apply these nutritional recommendations and tactics for meal frequency, portion control, and hydration into your daily life as we move through this book. Together, they serve as the foundation of a wholesome diet for seniors. In order to create your road to radiant health in your senior years, let's dig deeper.

CHAPTER 3

SUPERFOODS FOR SENIORS

Superfoods are the colourful threads in the ageing tapestry that can make your older years more attractive, resilient, and active. This section, "Superfoods for Seniors," is your ticket to a world of nutrient-dense treats that can help you age gracefully and improve the quality of your life. Here, we'll delve into the essence of antioxidant-rich foods to keep your skin looking young, learn about nutrition for healthy bones and joints, and examine the potential of brain-boosting superfoods to sustain cognitive function.

Antioxidant-Rich Foods for Aging Gracefully

Our bodies continually struggle with the effects of oxidative stress as we travel through the ageing process. During this process, unstable chemicals called free radicals can harm cells and hasten ageing. Nature's defenders, antioxidants, step in to assist combat harmful free radicals and defend your cells.

Foods high in antioxidants are your allies in this fight against the passing of time. They are brimming with vitamins, minerals, and phytonutrients that snuff out inflammation, promote the health of your cells, and maintain the radiance of your skin. These foods consist of:

1. Berries: Berries like blueberries, strawberries, and raspberries are bursting with antioxidants like vitamin C and anthocyanins that fight oxidative stress and improve skin health.

2. Leafy Greens: Antioxidants like lutein and zeaxanthin, which are abundant in spinach, kale and Swiss chard, promote eye health and eyesight as you age.

3. Nuts and Seeds: Rich in vitamin E and good

fats that hydrate your skin and shield your cells are almonds, walnuts, flaxseeds, and chia seeds.

4. Dark Chocolate: Flavonoids and other antioxidants found in premium dark chocolate with a cocoa level of 70% or higher improve heart health and promote cognitive function.

5. Tea: Both black tea and green tea include theaflavins, an antioxidant with antioxidant characteristics that supports general health.

You may age gracefully by include these antioxidant-rich foods in your diet on a regular basis since they protect your cells, lessen inflammation, and keep your skin looking young.

Foods for Strong Bones and Joints

For mobility and a high standard of living as you age, you need strong bones and joints. Your food decisions become increasingly more crucial for sustaining bone health as your body evolves. You can use the following meals as allies in this effort:

1. Dairy and fortified plant-based milks are excellent providers of calcium and vitamin D,

which are necessary for preserving bone health and density.

2. Fatty Fish: Fish rich in omega-3 fatty acids that improve joint health and reduce inflammation include salmon, sardines, and mackerel.

3. Leafy Greens: Bok choy, spinach, and collard greens are great providers of calcium and vitamin K, both of which are essential for strong bones.

4. Nuts and Seeds: Minerals like magnesium and phosphorus, which support healthy bones, are present in almonds, chia seeds, and flaxseeds.

5. Legumes and tofu: These plant-based sources of protein and minerals promote bone health and could serve as a meat-free protein substitute.

6. Oranges and citrus fruits are high in vitamin C, which helps to encourage the development of collagen for healthy joints.

You can nourish your bones and joints and make sure they are strong and robust throughout your golden years by include these items in your diet.

Brain-Boosting Superfoods

The finest nutrition should be given to your brain, the jewel of your body, to maintain it flexible and youthful as you age. A variety of minerals found in several superfoods can boost memory, cognition, and overall brain health.

1. Fatty Fish: As previously indicated, fatty fish high in omega-3 fatty acids, including salmon, trout, and sardines, may help lower the risk of cognitive decline. Omega-3 fatty acids are crucial for maintaining brain function.

2. Berries: In particular, blueberries are well known for their capacity to enhance memory and cognitive function.

3. Leafy Greens: Kale, spinach, and collard greens are excellent sources of nutrients such as vitamin K, lutein, and folate, which are associated with cognitive health.

4. Nuts: Omega-3 fatty acids, antioxidants, and vitamin E found in walnuts in particular enhance brain health.

5. Turmeric, an antioxidant and anti-inflammatory

compound found in turmeric, may have neuroprotective effects.

These brain-boosting superfoods can help you maintain cognitive function and improve your general quality of life as you age. When consumed as a group, these foods have the power to improve your overall health, encourage healthy ageing, and nourishes your body, mind, and spirit as you enter your golden years. Here are some helpful hints to take advantage of them:

1. Fatty Fish:

- Grilled or Baked Fish: Grill or bake salmon, trout, or sardines with a sprinkle of herbs and lemon for flavour.
- Fish Tacos: To make fish tacos, use whole-grain tortillas, a delicious salsa, and leafy vegetables.
- Fish Salad: To a salad of mixed greens, berries, and a light vinaigrette, add flakes salmon or trout.

2. Berries:

- For a wholesome and filling snack, combine Greek yoghurt with a bowl of mixed berries.
- Smoothies: For a cool smoothie, combine

blueberries, banana, spinach, and a little honey in a blender.
- Muesli with Berries: To add a splash of colour and flavour to your morning bowl of muesli, add a few berries.

3. Green smoothies with leafy greens.

- For a filling green smoothie, combine fruits like mango and pineapple with kale, spinach, or collard greens.
- Salads: Use a variety of greens to make robust salads, and top them with nuts, seeds, and a tasty dressing.
- Chopped leafy greens can be used to stir-fries or soups to boost their nutritional value.

4. Nuts:

- Add almond or walnut butter to a smoothie or spread it on whole-wheat bread.
- Make your own trail mix by combining different nuts, dried fruits, and dark chocolate chips.
- Salads: To provide a pleasing crunch, sprinkle chopped nuts on top of salads.

5. Turmeric:

- To make turmeric tea, soak turmeric powder in

hot water or milk for a few minutes.

- Curry meals: Use turmeric, a crucial component of many Indian and Asian recipes, to make curry meals.
- Roasted vegetables with turmeric: To add flavour and health benefits, sprinkle turmeric over the cooked vegetables.

Remember to talk to a doctor if you have any specific dietary limitations or health issues. These recommendations can assist seniors in incorporating superfoods into their regular diets, boosting overall and cognitive health in a tasty and engaging way.

CHAPTER 4

SPECIAL DIETS AND HEALTH CONDITIONS

This chapter, "Special Diets and Health Conditions," serves as your compass for navigating these threads in your later years. In the broad tapestry of health and nutrition, there are specific threads devoted to managing distinct health concerns. Here, we look into heart-healthy eating, diabetes management through nutrition, and specific diets adapted to common health issues.

Heart-Healthy Eating for Seniors

As you enter your golden years, eating heart-healthy foods should be your top priority. Seniors frequently worry about heart disease, and your diet has a big impact on your cardiovascular health.

Following are some essential guidelines for heart-healthy eating:

- Favour Healthy Fats: Choose the unsaturated fats found in avocados, salmon, and other fatty fish instead of saturated fats. These fats can lower levels of harmful cholesterol and lower the chance of developing heart disease.

- Reduce your intake of foods high in saturated fats, such as red meat and full-fat dairy products. Limit Saturated and Trans Fats. Avert the trans fats that are frequently found in processed and fried foods.

- Increase your intake of fibre: Fiber-rich foods, such as whole grains, fruits, and vegetables, can help decrease cholesterol and improve heart health.

- Lower Your Sodium Intake: Consume less sodium to reduce your risk of high blood pressure and heart disease. Reducing processed and high-sodium foods is a necessary step in this approach.

- Lean Proteins: To cut back on saturated fat intake, choose lean protein sources such tofu, poultry, fish, and legumes.

- Portion Control: Be mindful of the size of your portions to prevent overeating, which can lead to weight gain and heart health problems.

By establishing these heart-healthy eating routines, you can improve your cardiovascular health and reduce your risk of developing heart disease in your later years.

Managing Diabetes through Diet

Diet is crucial in preserving blood sugar levels and general health for people with diabetes who are managing the disease in their later years. Your quality of life can be improved and issues can be avoided with proper diet.

Following are some dietary recommendations for regulating diabetes:

- Carbohydrate Control: Keep an eye on and manage your consumption of carbs, concentrating on complex carbohydrates and avoiding foods with a high glycemic index.

- Balanced Meals: To help control blood sugar levels, prepare balanced meals that contain lean meats, healthy grains, and lots of non-starchy veggies.

- Fiber-Rich Foods: To slow down the absorption of sugar and enhance blood sugar control, include fiber-rich foods like whole grains, legumes, and vegetables in your diet.

- Choose unsaturated fats, which are present in nuts, seeds, and olive oil, to promote heart health.

- Consistent Meal Timing: Controlling portions and meal timing can help reduce blood sugar levels.

- Monitoring and Modifying: Regularly check your blood sugar levels and, in agreement with your healthcare provider, modify your diet as necessary.

A well-balanced diet and effort are necessary for managing diabetes with nutrition. You can improve blood sugar control and lower your risk of complications from diabetes by following these recommendations.

Special Diets for Common Health Concerns

Common health issues frequently call for specialised diets designed to meet particular requirements. It's critical to adjust your diet in accordance with any dietary restrictions brought on by other medical disorders, such as high blood pressure, digestive problems, or other concerns.

Numerous common health issues, including diabetes and heart disease, may call for particular diets. These could consist of:

1. High Blood Pressure (Hypertension): Blood pressure can be controlled with a low-sodium diet. Concentrate on eating natural, unadulterated foods and cut back on salt.

2. Osteoporosis: Bone health depends on a diet

high in calcium and vitamin D. Leafy greens, dairy products, and fortified foods can all be helpful.

3. Arthritis: Consuming foods that are anti-inflammatory, such as fatty fish, olive oil, and vibrant fruits and vegetables, will help reduce the symptoms of arthritis.

4. Digestive Problems: Low-fiber, readily digestible meals may be beneficial for seniors with digestive problems. Peeled and cooked fruits and vegetables may be simpler to digest.

While these dietary suggestions are typically good, it's vital to keep in mind that everyone has different demands. When addressing particular health issues, speaking with a certified dietician or other healthcare expert is strongly advised. To improve senior health and wellbeing, they can offer individualised advice and nutritional regimens.

The importance of identifying common health issues and designing diets to address them is emphasised in this chapter. Seniors can traverse their golden years with improved health and a higher quality of life by embracing specialised diets deliberately and proactively.

CHAPTER 5

COOKING AND MEAL PREPARATION

The culinary skills of cooking and food preparation will form the basis of your long-term nutritional quest. This chapter, "Cooking and Meal Preparation," will help you navigate this crucial step in your pursuit of vibrant health by examining the world of simple and nourishing recipes for seniors, providing helpful advice for cooking for one or two, delving into the art of meal planning and grocery shopping, and exploring the world of easy and nutritious recipes for children.

Easy and Nutritious Recipes for Seniors

Nutrition and simplicity are the two guiding principles when it comes to cooking for senior citizens. It is not only feasible but also necessary to maintain a balanced diet to prepare meals that are both quick and nourishing. Here are some guidelines to keep in mind:

- One-Pot Wonders: Recipes that can be produced in a single pot or skillet are quick to prepare and require little cleanup. Consider nourishing, comforting soups, stews, and stir-fries.

- Slow Cooker Magic: Slow cookers are a godsend for elders. You can prepare the ingredients in the morning and have a nice, filling meal waiting for you when you get home. It's the best method for creating nutrient-dense soups, tender meats, and vegetable-heavy dishes.

- Batch cooking: You can save time and effort on subsequent days by preparing larger servings and storing leftovers. Additionally, it guarantees you have quick, wholesome options when you don't feel like cooking.

- Simple Salads: A healthy salad doesn't need to be difficult to prepare. Salads made of leafy greens, vegetables, and a protein source like grilled chicken or chickpeas are a good idea. For flavour, drizzle a simple vinaigrette over top.

Smoothies are an easy and quick method to include a range of nutrients in a single meal. Combine fruits, leafy greens, yoghurt, and a protein source for a filling and readily absorbed meal.

Cooking for One or Two: Practical Tips

Cooking for just one or two people might be difficult for many elders. When you're used to cooking for a larger family, it could seem overwhelming to make a whole supper. Here are some helpful hints to make the procedure easier to handle:

- Prepare Smaller Portions: Tailor dishes to your preferences and avoid preparing large quantities. You can make fresh meals more frequently if you cook for fewer people.

- Freeze Extras: When preparing foods like soups or casseroles that freeze well, portion them into smaller servings and freeze the extras. You'll have quick, wholesome meals on hand in this manner for days when you don't feel like cooking.

- Make Use of Small Kitchen Appliances Toaster ovens, microwaves, and countertop grills are examples of small kitchen appliances that can speed up cooking. For making single or multiple portions, they are ideal.

- Use Convenience Foods Carefully: Convenience foods can save time, but you should be aware of their nutritional value. Make a healthy choice, such as pre-cut vegetables or canned beans, but watch out for added sugar or excessive salt.

- Fresh items: When preparing a meal for one or two people, try to use only fresh items. A nutritious dinner is built on a foundation of whole grains, fresh veggies, and lean proteins.

Meal Planning and Grocery Shopping

Making cooking and meal preparation a smooth part of your everyday routine requires effective grocery shopping and meal planning. Consider the following tactics:

- Weekly Meal Plans: Plan your meals for the following seven days, including breakfast, lunch, and dinner. This makes your shopping list more organised and guarantees you have the necessary ingredients.

- Use a shopping list every time you go shopping. Make a list of the ingredients you'll need for your scheduled meals and follow it. As a result, impulsive purchases are less likely.

- Frozen and Pantry Staples: Stock up on staples like canned veggies, nutritious grains, lean proteins, and frozen fruits to keep your freezer and pantry filled. You can add these components in place of some of your fresh ingredients.

- Shop During Off-Peak Hours: If you want to avoid crowds and make your shopping experience more convenient, think about going shopping during off-peak hours when the store is less crowded.

- Take into account internet shopping: Many grocery stores provide online shopping and delivery options, which can be advantageous if mobility is an issue.

By using these techniques, you may make meal preparation and cooking a productive and fun part of your daily schedule. It's an opportunity to use your culinary imagination while providing your body with scrumptious, healthy meals.

You will acquire the information and abilities necessary to make the most of this crucial component of your nutritional journey in your golden years as we continue our investigation of cooking and meal preparation. This chapter is your guide to welcoming cooking with open arms as a pleasurable and satisfying experience that improves your health and well-being.

Knowledge and Skills Required in Cooking and Meal Preparation

A valuable skill for seniors who want to keep their independence and health is cooking and food preparation. The following are the knowledge and abilities needed in this field:

Knowledge

1. Food Safety: In order to prevent foodborne

infections, it is essential to understand the fundamentals of food safety. This includes understanding of hygienic practises, temperature management, and food storage.

2. Nutrition: Creating balanced, healthy meals requires a basic understanding of nutrition. It is crucial to understand both macronutrients (carbohydrates, proteins, and fats) and micronutrients (vitamins and minerals).

3. Dietary Restrictions: Knowledge about dietary requirements, allergies, and specific medical conditions, such as diabetes, heart disease, or celiac disease, that may affect dietary choices.

4. Portion management: Maintaining a healthy weight and a balanced diet requires understanding portion sizes and the significance of portion management.

5. Culinary Skills: The ability to cook simply by chopping, sauté ing, boiling, roasting, and baking.

6. Flavour Profiles: Recognising various flavour profiles and learning how to balance sweet, salty, sour, acidic, bitter, and umami flavours to produce foods that are well-rounded.

1. Knife Skills: The capacity to use kitchen knives for dicing, chopping, and slicing securely and effectively.

2. The ability to prepare meals in advance while taking into consideration dietary needs and personal preferences.

3. Grocery Shopping: Making cost-effective choices for fresh, high-quality foods at the grocery store.

4. Reading recipes and comprehending them, including ingredient lists, conversions, and cooking directions.

5. Time management: Coordinating the cooking and preparation of various meal-related ingredients to guarantee that everything is ready at the same time.

6. Organisation: To work effectively and securely, a kitchen must be kept clean and organised.

7. Adaptation: The capacity to modify recipes to accommodate ingredient availability or dietary limitations.

8. Cooking Techniques: Expertise in a variety of cooking techniques, such as baking, grilling, broiling, steaming, and pan-frying.

9. Flavour Enhancement: The ability to employ seasonings, herbs, and spices to improve the flavour of food.

10. Appetisingly plating and displaying food so that it pleases the eyes as well as the palate.

11. Meal Storage: Recognising safe and effective methods for keeping leftovers.

12. Problem-Solving: The capacity to troubleshoot and modify when circumstances in the kitchen do not go as expected.

13. Tasting food: Experimenting with different flavours to learn how to taste food and adjust spice as necessary.

14. Kitchen Safety: Maintaining kitchen safety, which includes managing hot objects, preventing cross-contamination, and fire safety.

15. Cleaning Skills: The capacity to tidy up

after preparing food, including washing dishes, utensils, and kitchen surfaces.

It is possible for seniors to retain a pleasant and healthy diet, support their independence, and perhaps find a new enthusiasm for cooking during their golden years by learning and developing these knowledge and skills.

CHAPTER 6

STAYING ACTIVE AND EATING RIGHT

The interplay between physical activity and nutrition is the canvas on which vivid health is painted in the mosaic of your senior years. This chapter, "Staying Active and Eating Right," examines the close relationship between these two factors and how weight control supports healthy ageing. Here, we examine the crucial relationship between physical activity and nutrition and reveal the keys to sustaining a healthy weight.

The Connection Between Physical Activity and Nutrition

On your journey to robust health, physical exercise and nutrition go hand in hand. Your body gets the energy it needs from the food you eat to carry out daily activities and maintain general health. Your energy needs are influenced by the amount of energy you use up when exercising. For your health to be at its best, it is essential to comprehend this link.

The relationship between nutrition and exercise is as follows:

- Energy Balance: Exercise contributes to maintaining a healthy level of energy. You could put on weight if you eat more calories than you burn. On the other hand, you might lose weight if you exercise more than you eat in a day. Maintaining a healthy weight requires striking the correct balance.

- Improved Nutrient Utilisation: Physical exercise improves your body's ability to use nutrients. This is particularly significant for absorbing vitamins and minerals that are required for bone health, like calcium and vitamin D.

- Metabolic Health: Regular exercise helps maintain a healthy metabolism, enabling your body to consume and utilise nutrients efficiently.

- Appetite Control: Exercise can alter your appetite, making it simpler to regulate portion sizes and make nutritious meal selections.

- Muscle Maintenance: Resistance training and strength training are essential for maintaining muscle mass. Muscle loss as we age is a typical worry, and preserving it promotes general health and mobility.

Your well-being and quality of life will improve as you age if you incorporate regular physical activity and a healthy diet into your daily routine.

Weight Management and Healthy Aging

A key component of healthy ageing is weight management, which is directly related to both physical activity and diet. In addition to supporting your physical health, maintaining a healthy weight also promotes lifespan and mental clarity. Several important factors for managing weight are listed below:

- Balanced Diet: A healthy weight can only be attained and maintained with a diet that is both well-balanced and meets your nutritional demands. Put an emphasis on nutrient-dense foods and portion control.

- Physical activity: Regular exercise is essential for weight management. This includes both cardiovascular and strength training. It promotes a healthy metabolism, lean muscle growth, and calorie burning.

- Mindful Eating: Paying attention to your eating patterns can help you control your portions and prevent overeating. Savour each bite, pay attention to your hunger and fullness indicators, and stay focused on your food.

- Hydration: Keeping a healthy weight requires proper hydration. Sometimes people confuse hunger with thirst. Water might help you regulate your hunger before meals.

- Sleep and Stress: Maintaining a healthy weight requires getting enough sleep and managing stress. Stress and sleep deprivation both contribute to weight growth. Give importance to these well-being facets.

- Consultation: If you need individualised advice on weight control, think about speaking with a licenced dietitian or other healthcare expert.

There are no fad diets or false expectations in weight control. Finding a dependable and balanced approach to your diet and exercise that improves your health and wellbeing is the goal. You can enjoy your golden years with vitality and energy by keeping a healthy weight.

Creating a Harmonious Relationship between Physical Activity, Nutrition and Weight Management

For overall health and well-being, especially in the later years of life, it is crucial to establish a harmonious link between physical activity, nutrition, and weight management. Here is how these components might complement one another:

1. Physical Activity:

Benefits:

- Regular exercise promotes cardiovascular health, builds bones and muscles, and improves flexibility.
- By raising metabolism and burning calories, it helps with weight management.
- Exercise improves cognitive function and mental health by lowering stress.
- It can enhance balance, mobility, and lower the risk of falls, all of which are vital for senior citizens.

How to Achieve Harmony:

- To keep motivated, pick activities you enjoy, such as walking, swimming, dancing, or yoga.
- Aim for a balance between flexibility, strength training, and aerobic exercise.
- Gradually increase the duration and intensity of your workouts to put more stress on your body and develop strength.
- To develop a personalised workout programme that is both safe and effective, speak with a healthcare practitioner or a fitness professional.

2. Nutrition:

Benefits:

- A well-balanced diet promotes weight management and offers vital nutrients for overall health.
- A senior's ability to retain bone density and muscular mass depends on their diet.
- It aids with digestion and maintains gastrointestinal health.
- Emotional health and cognitive performance can both be improved by a balanced diet.

How to Achieve Harmony:

- Make eating a diet high in fruits, vegetables, whole grains, lean proteins, and healthy fats a priority.
- Use portion control to limit calorie consumption.
- Keep hydrated by consuming adequate water throughout the day.
- To design a customised meal plan that meets your nutritional needs, think about speaking with a trained dietitian.

3. Weight Management:

Benefits:

- Retaining a healthy weight lowers your risk of developing chronic illnesses and improves your quality of life in general.
- Losing weight can reduce joint pain and increase mobility.
- It promotes cardiovascular health and reduces the risk of diabetes and high blood pressure.
- Achieving and maintaining a healthy weight can increase body confidence and self-esteem.

How to Achieve Harmony:

- Establish a calorie balance by keeping track of how many calories you are consuming and using up through exercise.
- Establish reasonable goals for weight loss that take into account your age, health, and specific requirements.
- Regularly weigh yourself and take measurements to keep tabs on your progress.
- When necessary, get assistance from a medical expert, a qualified dietician, or a personal trainer.

By realising how closely these factors are related, we can attain balance between exercise, nutrition, and weight management. You can live a full and active life throughout your golden years by using a holistic approach, in which these elements support and enhance one another for your general wellbeing.

CHAPTER 7

OVERCOMING NUTRITION CHALLENGES

The fabric of your golden years may occasionally contain nutrition problems. This chapter, "Overcoming Nutrition Challenges," will serve as your road map for dealing with these problems politely and intelligently. In this article, we'll look at ways to support digestive health, deal with changes in appetite and taste, and comprehend how vitamins for seniors can help you stay healthy overall.

Promoting Digestive Health

As we become older, our need for digestive health grows. It is the foundation of our entire health. Your body will properly absorb nutrients from the meals you eat if you have a healthy digestive tract. To encourage digestive health, consider the following tactics:

- Include Foods High in Fibre: Include foods high in fibre, such as whole grains, legumes, fruits, and vegetables. Constipation can be avoided and supported by regular bowel movements.

- Probiotics: Foods with probiotics, such as yoghurt, kefir, and fermented vegetables, support a balanced population of good bacteria in the stomach and improve digestion.

- Hydration: For a good digestion, one must drink enough water. You can keep your digestive system running smoothly and soften stools by drinking water.

- Chew Your Food: Give your food a good, long chew. The first step in digestion is chewing, which also lessens the strain on your digestive system.

- Regular Meals: To promote your body's natural digestion pattern, keep regular meal times. Issues like indigestion and acid reflux may be avoided in this way.

- Limit Trigger Foods: If specific foods, including spicy or oily foods, make you bloated or uncomfortable, think about lowering your intake.

Addressing Changes in Appetite and Taste

As we become older, our tastes and appetites often change, which might provide special nutritional concerns. How to navigate these changes is as follows:

- Small, Frequent Meals: If you find it difficult to eat large meals due to a decreased appetite, think about eating smaller, more frequent meals and snacks to make sure you're still getting the nourishment you need.

- Flavorful Cooking: To make your meals more

appetising, experiment with herbs, spices, and healthful seasonings. This may be used to make up for shifts in taste perception.

- Texture Modification: Change the texture of your food if chewing or swallowing is becoming tough. To do this, you might puré e, mash, or choose foods that are softer and easier to chew.

- Appreciate Social Meals: Eating with friends and family can make meals more enjoyable. Eating with others can increase appetite and enhance general wellbeing.

- Drink Plenty of Water: Dehydration has an impact on taste and appetite. To support your taste perceptions, make sure you are sufficiently hydrated.

- Speak with a Healthcare Professional: To rule out underlying medical concerns and get individualised advice, speak with a healthcare professional if appetite or taste changes are severe and persistent.

The Role of Supplements for Seniors

Seniors who have particular nutritional needs may benefit from supplements. While a well-balanced diet is often the best way to get all the nutrients you need, some people might benefit from taking supplements. The following are important things to remember:

- Vitamin D: In order to preserve bone health, many seniors need vitamin D pills, especially if they get little sun exposure.

- Vitamin B12: To avoid deficits, senior citizens who follow vegetarian or vegan diets may need vitamin B12 supplements.

- Calcium: Supplements can assist bone health if you struggle to satisfy your calcium requirements through diet alone.

- Omega-3 Fatty Acids: Omega-3 dietary supplements are good for the heart and the brain.

- Multivitamins: For people on restrictive diets or who have trouble ingesting a range of foods, a daily multivitamin can fill in nutrient gaps.

- Consultation: To ascertain your individual requirements and guarantee safety and efficacy, speak with a healthcare professional or certified dietician before taking supplements.

Overcoming nutrition difficulties in your golden years is a credit to your adaptation and resilience. You can overcome these difficulties with grace and embrace vibrant health and well-being by putting these techniques for enhancing digestive health, dealing with changes in appetite and taste, and taking supplements into account.

CHAPTER 8

DINING OUT AND SOCIAL EATING

Social interaction and going out to eat are important aspects of life that become even more important as you get older. This chapter, "Dining Out and Social Eating," offers advice on how to make smart restaurant food selections and offers tips for negotiating family dinners and social gatherings with grace and wellbeing in mind.

Making Healthy Choices When Eating Out

Eating out may be a fun experience because it gives you a break from cooking and an opportunity to try new foods. With so many tempting options available, it also brings the problem of making good decisions. The following tips can assist you in keeping a healthy diet even when dining out:

- Examine the Menu Before You Go: A lot of restaurants now offer online menus. Use this opportunity to prepare your dinner and choose healthier options before you arrive.

- Opt for lower Portions: Check the menu for things with lower serving sizes, or think about having an appetiser for your main course.

- Choose Grilled or Baked Dishes: Opt for grilled, baked, or roasted dishes rather than fried or deep-fried ones. As a result, fewer harmful fats are consumed.

- Request Meal Modifications: Don't be afraid to request changes to your meal. Request whole-grain bread instead of white, a double portion of veggies, or a salad with the dressing on the side, for instance.

- Share Desserts: By splitting a sweet treat with your dining partner, you can indulge in a sweet delight without going overboard.

- Portion Control: Pay attention to serving sizes. When your meal is ready, you can ask for a to -go box and reserve a piece for later.

- Remain Hydrated: To help you manage portion sizes and keep hydrated, drink water throughout the meal.

- Limit Alcohol: If you prefer to consume alcohol, do it sparingly and consider how it will affect your total calorie consumption.

- Engage in Mindful Eating: Take your time while eating, savour each bite, and pay attention to your hunger and fullness signs. You can prevent overeating by doing this.

Navigating Social Gatherings and Family Meals

In order to build relationships, celebrate life, and spend time with loved ones, social events and family meals are essential. Here are some tips for dealing with these situations while keeping your health and wellbeing in mind:

- Express Your Dietary Preferences: Before the event, let your host or family members know your dietary preferences and limits. This may make it easier for them to meet your demands.

- Volunteer to Help: If you're going to a potluck or family reunion, volunteer to bring a wholesome food that you like and can share with others.

- Serving tiny amounts of your favourite foods at social gatherings is a good way to practise portion control. savour the flavours without going overboard.

- Talk to People: Talking with loved ones and friends will help you slow down your eating rate and avoid overeating.

- Enjoy Without Guilt: Don't feel guilty about indulging in special meals and treats. A healthy relationship with food includes the occasional excesses, so keep that in mind.

- Put the People You're With First: While food

plays a big role in social gatherings, the people you're with should come first. Take advantage of the relationships and time spent together.

- Stay Active: Include exercise in your daily regimen to counteract any indulgences you may have at social occasions.

By putting these tactics into practise, you may enjoy eating out, enjoy socialising with family and friends, and still maintain your health and wellbeing. These opportunities provide a chance to feed both your body and your soul.

CHAPTER 9

TRACKING YOUR NUTRITION

Maintaining good health in your senior years requires careful attention to your diet. In order to make sure that your nutritional needs are satisfied, this chapter, "Tracking Your Nutrition," offers insight into the advantages of food journals and apps as tools for self-evaluation and communication with healthcare specialists.

The Benefits of Food Journals and Apps

A valuable tool for self-evaluation and sustaining a healthy diet is food journaling. Food diaries and mobile applications made for this purpose have the following advantages:

- Greater Awareness: Food monitoring makes you more aware of what you're consuming, which is beneficial if you have particular dietary objectives or limits.

- Recognising Patterns: You can spot patterns in your eating behaviour over time. This can assist you in understanding when and why you choose particular foods.

- Portion Control: Keeping track of your dietary intake will help you control portion sizes and avoid overeating.

- Monitoring Nutrient Intake: Apps and food journals frequently offer nutrient breakdowns that let you check whether you're getting the daily recommended amounts of vitamins, minerals, and macronutrients.

- Accountability: Being aware that you are

tracking your meals might help you be more responsible and motivate you to choose healthier foods.

- Goal Setting: You can set precise dietary objectives and monitor your progress towards attaining them by keeping a food journal.

- Assessment of Allergies or Sensitivities: Keeping a thorough food journal can help you and your healthcare practitioner find potential triggers if you believe you have allergies or sensitivities to certain foods.

Collaboration with Healthcare Professionals

A crucial part of managing your nutrition is working with medical professionals, especially if you have particular health issues or dietary restrictions:

- Registered dietitians and nutritionists can provide individualised advice based on your dietary requirements and health objectives. They can assist you in developing a customised food plan and ensuring that you are fulfilling your unique needs.

- Medical professionals: Your general practitioner or a specialist can handle any health issues that can affect your nutritional requirements. They can offer suggestions for using nutrition to control or enhance your health.

- Pharmacists: If you take drugs, your chemist can provide advice on how particular foods and supplements may interact with your medications as well as information on whether you should avoid or recommend them.

- Allergists: An allergist can detect allergies or sensitivities and offer detailed advice on avoiding triggers and making dietary changes.

- Registered nurses: Nurses are essential in keeping an eye on your general health and might recommend dietary adjustments to promote your wellbeing.

- Geriatric specialists: These healthcare professionals are trained to address the special health requirements of older persons, including dietary issues associated with ageing.

Working with medical professionals will help you

make dietary decisions that are compatible with your health objectives and any existing medical issues. These professionals can offer the direction you need to successfully manage the challenges of nutrition in your later years.

Utilizing Food Journals and Apps to Track Your Nutrition Effectively

You may track your diet, make wise decisions, and reach your health and wellness objectives during your senior years with the help of food journals and smartphone applications. Here is a step-by-step instruction on how to use them:

1. Pick the Right Tool: Opt for a food diary or mobile app that fits your requirements and tastes. Popular choices include Lose It!, Cronometer, and MyFitnessPal. These applications include tools for goal-setting, nutrient tracking, and food databases.

2. Establish Specific Goals: Choose what you hope to accomplish with your nutrition tracking. Common objectives include maintaining a healthy weight, treating particular health issues, or simply eating a balanced diet. Make sure

your objectives are Time-bound, Specific, Measurable, Achievable, and Relevant. For instance, "I want to lose 10 pounds in three months by reducing daily calorie intake."

3. Keep Track of Your Meals: Be meticulous in keeping track of each meal and snack you have. Include information about serving sizes, cooking techniques, and any sauces or condiments. The majority of applications have sizable food databases, making it simple to locate and record the foods you consume. Make sure the entries you choose are accurate.

4. Watch Portion Sizes: To precisely gauge how much food you consume, use measuring cups, a food scale, or other portion control tools. Your ability to gauge portion sizes will improve with practise, which will be especially useful when dining out.

5. Keep tabs on Nutrient Intake: Numerous applications offer nutrient breakdowns for your meals. Pay close attention to vital nutrients like fibre, protein, and minerals. Contrast your nutrient intake with your objectives. To make sure you're getting all the nutrients you need each day, modify your diet.

6. Keep a Record of Meal Timing: Note the times

that you eat your meals and snacks. By doing so, you can spot patterns in your eating behaviour and, if necessary, make improvements.

7. Include Hydration: Remember to record your drinks. Your whole health depends on drinking enough water.

8. Evaluate and Reflect: Schedule regular time to evaluate the information in your diary or app. Analyse your eating habits for patterns, places for development, and advancement towards your objectives. Consider the rationale behind your dietary decisions. Were they motivated by hunger, feelings, or other outside forces? Making better selections in the future can be aided by thinking back on your past decisions.

9. Modify and Set New Goals: Modify your diet as needed in light of your reflections and advancement. This could entail changing food selections, quantity levels, or scheduling of meals. Set new objectives as you reach your initial ones to keep enhancing your diet and general wellbeing.

10. Seek Advice: Consult with medical specialists or qualified dietitians for individualised advice and suggestions if you

have certain health problems, dietary limitations, or complicated nutritional demands.

11.   Maintain Consistency: To see results, you must continuously track your nutrition. Make it a regular part of your day-to-day routine.

12.   Embrace Flexibility: While keeping track of your nutrition is important, be accommodating and kind to yourself. A healthy relationship with food includes occasional indulgences and dietary changes.

You may properly manage your nutrition, keep on track with your health objectives, and have a vigorous and well-nourished existence during your golden years by meticulously using food journals and apps and sticking to these instructions.

Enhancing Golden Years with Healthcare-Backed Nutrition

In order to make sure that your dietary choices support your bright health and general well-being during your golden years, working with healthcare specialists is an essential first step. The following are the main advantages of this cooperation:

1. Customised Advice: Healthcare specialists, particularly licenced dietitians and nutritionists, can offer dietary guidance that is specifically catered to your needs, preferences, and medical problems. Whether it's treating a chronic disease, losing weight, or improving your general wellbeing, they can develop a customised nutrition plan that supports your unique health goals.

2. Disease Management: Dietary decisions are also important for seniors who are treating chronic illnesses like diabetes, heart disease, or osteoporosis. You can effectively treat these disorders with dietary adjustments with the assistance of healthcare specialists, lowering the risk of complications and raising your quality of life.

3. Nutritional Optimisation: Your dietary requirements may alter as you get older. For the best mix of vitamins, minerals, and macronutrients, you can optimise your nutrient intake with the aid of healthcare professionals. They are able to spot any deficits and suggest the proper dietary changes or supplementation.

4. Medication-Nutrient Interactions: A number of drugs may have an impact on the effectiveness or absorption of certain nutrients. To assist you get the most out of your therapy, healthcare providers might advise you on which meals or supplements to encourage or avoid based on your meds.

5. Management of Allergies and Sensitivities: Dealing with food allergies and sensitivities can be particularly difficult. To keep you safe and healthy, healthcare professionals such as allergists and dietitians can diagnose your condition and offer detailed instructions on allergy avoidance and dietary modifications.

6. Support for Digestive Health: For elderly people who are having digestive problems, medical practitioners can suggest dietary approaches to support gut health and treat illnesses like celiac disease or irritable bowel syndrome (IBS). They can suggest dietary modifications that improve your digestive health and relieve symptoms.

7. Holistic tackle: Healthcare experts tackle your health holistically. Along with your nutritional choices, they take into account other things including your level of physical activity, sleep, and stress management. This all-

encompassing viewpoint is crucial for general health and active ageing.

8. Accountability and inspiration: Regular check-ins with medical experts can help with accountability and inspiration. Your nutrition and wellness objectives can help keep you on track and help you achieve long-term success if you know you have continuing support and coaching.

9. Preventive Care: Working with medical experts enables preventive care. You can lower your risk of getting certain problems by proactively changing your diet and recognising potential health hazards early. This will eventually help you maintain your robust health.

10.   Knowledge and Confidence: Consulting with medical experts can provide you the information and assurance need to make wise food decisions. You can actively participate in your health and wellbeing during your senior years thanks to this empowerment.

To ensure that your food decisions support your vibrant health and general well-being throughout your golden years, communication with healthcare specialists is a crucial component. Their knowledge, individualised support, and all-encompassing strategy are excellent assets that can promote a long and healthy life.

CHAPTER 10

EMBRACING VIBRANT HEALTH IN YOUR GOLDEN YEARS

Embracing vibrant health as you approach your elderly years is a journey of self-care, happiness, and fulfilment. This chapter, "Embracing Vibrant Health in Your Golden Years," represents the pinnacle of your dietary research. Setting and accomplishing nutrition goals, mindful eating for emotional well-being, and embracing a senior lifestyle of vibrant health are all covered in this article.

Setting and Achieving Nutrition Goals

The first step to thriving health in your golden years is to clearly define your nutritional goals. Setting and accomplishing nutrition goals is essential, whether your goals are focused on managing your weight, improving your energy levels, or treating a particular health condition. This is how you do it:

- Establish Your Goals: Begin by outlining your nutritional objectives. Make sure that they are SMART goals— specific, measurable, achievable, relevant, and time-bound.

- Break Down the Goals: Separate your broad objectives into more specific, doable stages. Set reasonable monthly goals, for instance, if you want to reduce weight.

- Make a nutrition plan. Keeping your goals in mind, make a nutrition plan that specifies the foods you should eat to help you reach your targets. To ensure a balanced diet, include a range of foods.

- Track Your Progress: Track your food consumption and keep an eye out for changes in your health or well-being to determine how well you are doing. If necessary, modify your plan.

- Maintain Accountability: Discuss your objectives with a supportive friend or relative who can serve as your accountability partner. As an alternative, seek advice from a qualified dietician or other medical expert.

- Honour Milestones: Honour your accomplishments along the path. Celebrate when you reach smaller checkpoints on the way to your main objective.

Mindful Eating and Emotional Well-being

By practising mindful eating, you can improve both your emotional and relationship with food. It entails eating with awareness and being present during meals. Here are some tips for mindful eating:

- Savour Each meal: Enjoy the flavours and textures of each meal slowly. You can enjoy your food more and avoid overeating by taking your time when eating.

- Listen to Your Body: Be aware of your body's

signals of hunger and fullness. Eat only when you are hungry, and only until you are full.

- Remove Distractions: Avoid using devices like smartphones, televisions, or computers while eating. You may concentrate on your food's sensory experience when you eat without interruptions.

- Select Nutrient-Dense Foods: Choose meals that are high in nutrients. By doing this, you can eat and fuel your body at the same time.

- Develop an Attitude of Gratitude: Take a moment to reflect on how much work it took to prepare the food on your plate and how much nourishment it offers.

- Awareness of Emotional Eating: Recognise your emotional eating habits. Look for healthy coping mechanisms if you frequently turn to food to deal with stress, boredom, or other emotions.

A Senior Lifestyle of Vibrant Health

In addition to eating, there are other components of a senior lifestyle that promote vigorous health:

- Exercise: Continue to lead an active lifestyle. Exercise regularly according to your ability and interests. It promotes emotional wellbeing in addition to physical wellness.

- Social Relationships: Develop and preserve social connections. Promoting mental health and a sense of belonging through interactions with friends, family, and your community.

- Mental Stimulation: Exercise your brain by reading, doing puzzles, or picking up new skills. For healthy cognitive function, mental activity is essential.

- Emotional Resilience: Develop emotional resilience by using stress-reduction tactics like deep breathing exercises or meditation.

- Routine Health Checkups: Be sure to get frequent health screenings. A senior lifestyle that is full of vitality and health depends on early detection and prevention.

- Positivity: Keep your view on life upbeat. To improve your wellbeing, embrace joy, laughter, and a sense of purpose.

You'll discover that robust health is not just about the food you eat, but also about a holistic approach to well-being as you embrace it in your golden years. This chapter offers advice on how to develop a senior lifestyle that is full of health and vitality, practise mindful eating for emotional well-being, and plan and meet nutrition objectives.

CONCLUSION

YOUR PATH TO VIBRANT HEALTH IN YOUR GOLDEN YEARS

Your investigation of how to embrace the golden years with nutrition, energy, and wellbeing through "Nutrition for Golden Years: A Senior's Guide to Vibrant Health" has been your adventure. We've travelled a thorough route through the following chapters, each of which provides insightful information and direction:

1. Needs in Nutrition vary with Age: Be aware that your body's metabolism and nutrient absorption vary as you become older. To support your changing health, modify your diet as necessary.

2. Important Nutrients for Senior Health: For overall senior health, give calcium, vitamin D, B vitamins, and fibre top priority.

3. Senior-Friendly Nutritional Recommendations: Build a nutritious diet for seniors by adhering to rules like moderation with portions, diversity, and balance.

4. Hydration Matters: Maintaining proper hydration is crucial for maintaining physical and mental health as you age.

5. Superfoods for Healthy Ageing: Include foods high in antioxidants, things that support bone and joint health, and foods that stimulate the brain in your diet.

6. Heart-Healthy Eating: To maintain cardiovascular health, emphasise a heart-healthy diet rich in lean proteins, whole grains, and unsaturated fats.

7. Dietary Control of Diabetes: Control diabetes by watching your carbohydrate consumption and selecting complex carbohydrates.

8. Special Diets for Health Concerns: Particular diets, such as those that are low in sodium or purines, can effectively address common health problems.

9. Efficient Cooking and Meal Preparation: Make meal preparation simple by using quick, wholesome recipes, modifying them for smaller households, and effectively planning meals.

10. Supplements to exercise Nutrition: A good diet and regular exercise together promote overall wellbeing.

11. Weight management: Keeping your weight in check is crucial for avoiding age-related health problems and promoting healthy ageing.

12. Encouraging Digestive Health: For a healthy digestive tract, prioritise fibre, probiotics, and hydration.

13. Take Care of Changing Preferences: Experiment with various flavours and textures

to take care of Changing Appetite and Taste.

14.   Supplements May Be Required: To fill in nutritional deficits, supplements such as calcium and vitamin D may be required.

15.   Dining Out Wisely: Review menus, use portion control, and make conscious decisions when eating out to make healthy choices.

16.   Navigating Social Eating: Be careful of your food choices while dining out and let others know what you prefer to eat.

17.   A benefit of food journals and apps is that they help measure nutritional intake and raise awareness of eating patterns.

18.   Collaboration with Healthcare specialists: Seek out individualised counsel from healthcare specialists to manage particular health issues or dietary limitations.

19.   Setting and Achieving Nutritional Goals: Establish SMART nutritional objectives, make a nutrition plan, and track your development to keep up a balanced diet.

20.   Mindful Eating and Emotional Well-being: Develop a mindful eating habit, enjoy every

mouthful, pay attention to your body's cues, and address emotional eating for a healthier connection with food.

21.   A Senior Lifestyle of Vibrant Health: Beyond diet, maintain an active lifestyle, social contacts, mental stimulation, emotional resilience, routine health examinations, and a positive outlook for general well-being in your senior years.

These important insights offer seniors a road map for navigating their senior years with assurance, embracing vigorous health, and savouring the pleasures of life with informed food decisions.

The information you've learned in these chapters has given you the skills you need to prioritise your health, make wise eating decisions, and feed both your body and soul. As you reach the finish line of this trip, keep in mind that maintaining vibrant health into your senior years requires a lifetime commitment. It's about enjoying the trip, marking significant anniversaries, and continuing to learn and advance.

The years of wisdom, vigour, and delight are in your

golden years. This book's pages serve as a gentle reminder that your diet has a significant impact on how you experience this priceless stage of life. It's important to enjoy the flavours, cherish the experiences, and treat your body with love and respect in addition to eating to live.

May the joy of a life well lived, the accumulation of your wisdom, and your strong health be a testament to your golden years. Continue to fuel your body, mind, and soul, and make each meal a reason to celebrate this amazing journey.

ADDITIONAL RESOURCES

A selection of helpful resources is provided below to help you on your way to enjoying strong health well into your golden years:

1. Books:

   - ➤ "Healthy Aging: A Lifelong Guide to Your Physical and Spiritual Well-Being" by Andrew Weil, M.D.
   - ➤ "The Longevity Diet" by Valter Longo, Ph.D.
   - ➤ "The Blue Zones Kitchen" by Dan Buettner.

2. Websites:

   - ➤ [National Institute on Aging

(NIA)](https://www.nia.nih.gov/): Offers a wealth of information on aging, health, and nutrition.
➤ [American Heart Association](https://www.heart.org/): Provides resources on heart-healthy eating for seniors.

3. Mobile Apps:

➤ MyFitnessPal: A popular app for tracking nutrition and exercise.
➤ Cronometer: A tool for detailed nutrient tracking.
➤ Lose It!: Helps with tracking calories and setting weight management goals.

4. Nutrition and Cooking Blogs:

➤ [EatingWell](https://www.eatingwell.com/): Offers healthy recipes and nutrition tips.
➤ [The Kitchn](https://www.thekitchn.com/): Provides cooking inspiration and tips.

5. Social Support Groups:

➤ Local senior centers or community groups

often host nutrition and wellness programs.
➤ Online forums and social media groups can connect you with others on a similar health journey.

6.   Registered   Dietitians   and   Healthcare Professionals:

➤ Consult with a registered dietitian or healthcare provider for personalized advice.

7. Exercise and Physical Activity Programs:**

➤ Consider joining local fitness classes, yoga groups, or walking clubs.
➤ SilverSneakers (for eligible Medicare beneficiaries) offers fitness programs and resources.

8.   Mental   Health   and   Stress   Management Resources:

➤ Explore meditation apps and programs.
➤ Consider local support groups or therapy sessions.

9. Continuing Education Programs:

> Local universities or online platforms offer courses on nutrition, cooking, and wellness.

10. Senior-Centric Organizations:

> Organizations like AARP provide resources and guidance on senior health and well-being.

11. Government Health Agencies:

> Visit websites of health agencies like the [CDC] (https://www.cdc.gov/) for valuable health information.

These resources can serve as valuable tools, references, and support systems for your journey toward vibrant health in your golden years. Remember to choose the resources that align with your specific health goals and preferences.

ABOUT THE AUTHOR

Grace Ben-Council is a fierce supporter of the health and wellbeing of senior citizens. Grace has spent years researching and imparting her knowledge to elders and their families. Grace has a background in nutrition and a strong dedication to supporting robust ageing. She thinks that everyone should be able to live happy and healthy lives into their later years.

In "Nutrition for Golden Years: A Senior's Guide to Vibrant Health," Grace blends her knowledge of nutrition with her commitment to offering seniors who want to make informed dietary decisions practical advice. She firmly believes that living a full and active life should be possible at any age.

Contact Information

For inquiries, speaking engagements, or collaboration opportunities, you can reach Jane Smith at:

Email: gracebencouncil@gmail.com

Phone: +234-906-211-3219

Feel free to contact Grace for any questions, feedback, or to explore opportunities for enhancing senior health and well-being.